Whirl Away Girl

Whirl Away Girl

Tricia Johnson

atmosphere press

Table of Contents

Distress

Emergence

Symptomatic

Fatigue

Fatigue
There should be a better word
Something more descriptive
Tiredness that steals in mid-sip coffee and forces your head flat
    on counter?
Tiredness that stops you in your tracks and screams
Sit NOW!
Lay down NOW!
If you don't
I will force you by simply stopping, unmoving, unbending

It strikes so many ways, so many times
Mid-shower, mid-sentence, mid-walk
Writing
Sitting
Walking
Cleaning, interrupting activity, for non-activity
There is no pushing through it
There is no way around

You are riding in a car and its weight slides in
and down your body
Your hands too heavy to knit
Your head too heavy to raise and no words or thoughts exist

It joins you for parties, mid-laugh, mid-thought
It glazes your eyes to a far off place
You visit more often than not

It is heavy, slow-motion drowning in fog
Trying to swim in jet black tar
That no one seems to feel but you
You are not air you are dense solid heavy
Wet clay earth stuck to the bottom of spring boots

Chasing My Tail

I liken my health to a dog chasing its tail
Each new symptom a circular path
Lupus? Virus? Side effect? Infection? Lupus?
Virus? Lupus? Side effect? Lupus?
Which is it? Which is first?
Which is treatable?
Chills with no fever
Burning joints
Clumsy fall of a ladder
Hurt your hand on a railing
I just want to lay down anywhere
Sweat patches in the night
Random circles
Awake awake miserable feeling awake
Hot cheeks flushing? That burning cheek feeling
Forgetful
What? Where? forgotten
Hard guilty sorry no energy
Did you tell me that?
Scared worried better yet?
Almost pass out in shower
Exhausted from showers
No jewelry
That takes energy
A trip for chicken equals couch time
Make dinner sit, sitting
Couldn't focus, not even knitting
Extra antibiotic for bacteria
3 more meds for yeast gone wild
Body fighting with what?
How does it fight with lowered immune system?
Is this the exhaustion?
Is it infection?
Is it medication?
Is it lupus?
No answers no clarity
I won't know they won't know

Does it matter, should it matter?
Obviously it does or I wouldn't write it
Frustration with chasing my tail

Morning

I am puffy swollen eyes
Red nose and cheeks
Rash covered chin tight burning itching
I am goobered up eyes
Dry scratchy, seeing unclearly
Clumsy, stiff joints
Moving slowly
Foggy brain
Morning lupus head

Hostile Takeover

I read frustration as criticism
I see worry as judgement
I want to conceal and smile
But really that is so unfair
To me
To them
Don't want to worry
Anyone including me
But here it is again
Unsavory health
Hostile stomach take over
That lets no one in or out
Gurgling ramparts
Combat with medicine missiles
That miss their target
And I am holed up here
Napping there
Swollen fingers, wrists
Death toxic breath mouth
Unmoving GI
Lying face down in vomit

Tearless

Chills and fingertips
Cold
Sad
Anxious
Jaw immobile clenched chipped teeth
Water eyes
Tears biological mechanical not for me
In the beginning, tears came often
And now I cannot find them
They are a lake of dryness
Until morning when the dam runs down
The corner of my eyes
Outside rivulets, swollen lid
Sigh

Disease in the Back Seat

In the tumble of life
Swirls the disease
Present in swollen right knee and ankle
Seen in bruises
Swollen eyes
Unbending knees, trapped in liquid
Upset stomach
Race to toilet
Three hours, still tired, nap

Hair flutters away in the breeze
Out the car window like bending string
Five, six, who knows how many more
Itchy skin, scalp, hands, ears, everywhere
Lurking in the back seat
Springing forth out my throat
Disease

Dealing with normal life, undealing
Swollen painful fingers
Shoulder aching pains, raw
Just live be normal
No, you are the goose, in the ducks
Running round and round
Lost in circles
Brain dizzy, falling down
Forgotten

Evening Decline

Nausea
Ill again
Fatigue
Floating, hovering mind
Numb gone blind
To things about and beyond
Unable to be present
Part of me gone
Out of touch of hand
No sleep
Spasm legs, ankles
Back pain
Bathroom break again
Up, up
Roll, turn, toss
Awake? To move?
Lie still and rest
Too warm?
Cold toes
Dark night, hurt
Cast outline unending decline
Hovering above the blue

Lupus

And the storm waves come again
Rash on chin, tight burning itchy stiff raised pustules of rash
Eyes swollen slanted crusty red-rimmed
Hair floating down tangled globs stuck to body, as shower
Stuck in all the wrong places
Leaving the scalp alone, forlorn, lonely
Knees with bubbles of fluid above, below, behind, stretched out circles
So oddly felt walking
Ankles, clicking, clunking, popping pain shoots up the center to the calf
Electrical nightmare hot
Freezing chills down spine can't feel toes or fingers
Shudder, curl smaller into fetal ball, sleep?
NO! freezing still, enough
Socks housecoat extra blanket hood fetal position once more
Shudder, shiver, sigh
Numb tingling lip, right lower, just side of center fluttering all day long
Butterflies landing?
Gas rolling, boiling, loud cramping diarrhea? nausea? stomach
Whoa sit down spinning
Slow down stop
Fatigue waves of fog, drifting in and out immobile, drifting mind sleep
Blue wave crush
In bed all morning
Shower
Bed
Lunch
Bed-finally moving
Food? who cares- medicines to be taken, food anyway
Yeast white clumpy masses everywhere, bottom to top, itchy angry,
    hard to swallow
Swollen lumps in mouth
Friendly, rash on neck and chest
Ever-present hassle unwanted guest
Hard bee-bee under skin hand unknown thing
Biopsy again needs to be gone
Warm hot rosy cheeks and nose burning
Puff-ball cheeks

11

Heart bumpy thump rhythm, airy skip flutter glide
Sweat down between breasts, running down face, back, thighs wet
    shirt drenched
Undergarments, vacuuming car
All in a day
All in a week
All of this, all, all of it me

Away

I feel the pull
To run and hide
Blankets tight curled body
Burrow down away from light
Rest pull the tangled mind back
To me, woven so far away

Reach for a dream pervasive as night
Cool as fog
Quiet as cold
Nowhere emotion bound
Nowhere flow, unfound
Eyes unblinking unseeing movement stopped
Shadow to page ink at play
The nowhere to here, to found on page

Travel to where?
A dream wish list?
I do not know
Always to beach- to water
To Pisces' love of sea
To land by sea
To shade

Far away? Close to home?
Worries gone?
A reprieve
Tentative so slowly written
Thoughts move out so carefully
Afraid to dream
To sort out
Fly-

Fearful demands of body
Disease steal
Family needs
Home needs

Always needs
Others not mine
Stifled by everything
Owning nothing
Sore stiff neck, stiff body
Tired body
Curl away to dream
Happy miles
Travel light
Warm wind
Half a world away

Nighttime Movement

Sleepy achy body
Knots in shoulders and neck
Knees hurting
Hurting in cold
In showers of snow
In storms brewing West of North
Coming
Inches
Piled high
Waiting rumors fly
Walk too much
Right knee cries
Lower back bright in the pain
Eyes sandy deep scratch swollen
Blind sand
See sand
Stare sand
The ocean miles away
Warm to hot water, pause take it away
Falling South
Gentle Earth filling but it stays
All of it
Wide eyes at night
Bathroom trips times 27
Head swirls
Hair shifts softly
Unable to sit still
Toe taps a rhythm
No one hears but me

Dry

Dry burning eyes
Cracked skin
Fine white lines playing across the skin

Dry burning eyes
Blurred with fatigue
Dry, brittle, parched me

Living in the sea of disease

Pieces

My cheeks have gone to rouge
Warm burning prickle
Nose across tops of cheeks
To temple just slightly lower
Burn shimmering burn
Burst across my face
Dancing its fearful meaning
Lupus singing shrilly
Familiar song
Cheeks circle bulbs of heat red warm hot
Low BP
Up and dizzy
Catch self
Catch bed
Catch wall
Catch arms out clothesline and all
Roller coaster head
Trying to walk a straight line
Swollen legs
Angry eyes
Gritty burning mad
Burning muscles
Traveling nerves twisting hurt
Neck to shoulder
Neck to shoulder adjust
Re-adjust
Pain
Range of motion stalling shrinking
Clumsy hands
Clumsy brain
Pieces of me not firing
Pieces of me fighting disease
Hurray!
Fighting and living moving
Functioning still

Treatments

Appointment Land

And on again
To appointment land
To hear the white-clad
Unanswered say
Clarity an elusive thread
Oh, the dread
The wait, the seat
The weight, the seat
The chat the guess
Begin what is next

Sad and Beat

The calm, the milk glass opaque
That swirls around my sight
As the latest cruel turn of health
Plagues my door, shadows
What late day-light remains, of the damp day

I have nowhere to hide
Unable to run
Rely on son to drive
As eyesight gone
Migraine danced in, an old song
Another doctor appointment to keep
And hurrah more medicine
A fool to not have done so before

Defeat in my voice in my movements
Just decide
I cannot
Just decide and I will do
I have no more critical thought
It's possible I simply do not care
The faded light is insipid in my soul
My colors have bled away

In this moment
In this now
Harsh lit paper-covered table room
Cubicle 8x8 maybe?
I am drained and leaving
To right this mind-
To encounter more bleak
Unable to obtain medicine anymore
This paper for that paper
To this number press 2
'Representative'
The drill the roll call
The wait

The check-in, the status
Another to solve resolve work out
This faded grey of me
She is sad and beat
Wishing on a miracle cure
Deluding herself it's possible, sad that it's unreasonable
Trying to be a warrior
As the milky murky water settles fills her blinky gritty eyes
Weights her person immobile
Hope has slid under the closed door and fled

Waiting on calls

Waiting
Wanting still
On hold
On life
On medical solutions
For the phone to ring
For it not to ring
For answers never coming
Cures unavailable
Side effects and more and beyond
Medicine again
Phone calls again
Still waiting
Waiting

Perfection Out of Reach

Very hard to stay impassive at doctors' appointments I want to be
  agreeable
I want to be rational
I want for so much
And it is slightly out of reach
To be impersonal when it is personal
To be rational in an irrational setting
My emotions boiling over in painful waves
Fear, anxiety, I am scared I place my future with you I want no
  mistakes
I want perfection in a very imperfect place
I don't want to make bad decisions or them to either I want the best
  probably
I want beyond the best
Exceeding it fully

Causeless

Emotions skitter on high alert
Tear prick eyes
Frustration
On lack of revelations
On definite recitations
Of cause

Probable cause
Not good enough
More appointments
Intolerable
More tests
Stress beyond capabilities

I need a moment
Or 25
To feel sunshine
To hear a cat purr
To hear my boys laughter
The taste of dark chocolate
A hug from my husband
I need peace

Instead
A chill runs down my legs
Up my back
Prickle my scalp
Low-grade fever
Feel ill
Unknown illness
Restless sleepless
Hurt nose
Cruel lullaby, sung off-key
In hoarse whisper

The Brush Off

Do you know?
Do I trust you?
Am I suspicious-yes
I am not the average person
I am not a quantifiable research statistic
I am not your other patients
I am not old or excessively young
I do not smoke
I am not overweight
Yes, yes, indeed my cardiomyopathy is slight
BUT, hey! I have cardiomyopathy
I have irregular heartbeats
I get short of breath
My heart beats so rapidly
I have to stop and sit
Or become dizzy and fall
But I pass your tests with 'Insignificant findings'
Yet a nurse remembers me 3 weeks later and asks
"Did you get your results?"
And her voice gives way to her worry and I am shocked into
immobility, pondering
She continues "take care of yourself, drink stay hydrated"
She holds my gaze directly, significantly
I am not dying this instant so really I am fine in the eyes of said sage
    doctors
All I ask is take me seriously
Me this woman in front of you
Who is sick and is trying to make it
Who is tired of runarounds
Who takes notes because she sees so many doctors
Who would like some relief from symptoms
Who is her own unique human being
Respect this human body that is me
And treat ME
Not your codes
Not your scales of numbers
Not your averages

ME
This beautiful creation with thoughts of futures and dreams
ME
This creative woman who loves passionately
ME
This woman who bravely marches on
For Heaven's sake
Please, please, treat me all 140 pounds, blue-eyed, blond hair with
     silver 5'7"
ME

New Doctor

Condescending eyes
Not liking being questioned
I'll admit I am scatterbrained, drift around in circles, this is what I do
My health it seems is complicated
By little insignificant complications
When added together become a 10-ton hammer
At times I feel marginalized and without respect
This doctor dance- kiss their toes so they continue to help
I scream inside NO YOU MORON YOU!!
Would you like to be me?
But maybe you have had a bad a day/night/year
And you're tired and cranky
And really want to stamp your diagnosis across my forehead
Treat it and move on
You're not into filling in questions just now
Check back next time
But I am hurting and hurt and could use some time focused on me
My uniqueness with definitive well thought out answers
That gives me peace
To continue on in hope
Not waiting around for the bottom to drop out
Preventative medicine
I am told, "if your ankles get 10x bigger or your knees or stomach
	then we will worry"
But alas what about the subtle types that can steal in the night
Slowly creep in and hurt you?
That is how this started!
There was no crash of mighty gong and voice chiming out "Look and
	see she is sick!"
Her heart with cardiomyopathy
But until I am dying
No need to fear
Ludicrous insane, ignorant man
I miss my old cardiologist
I miss the knowledge she shared
I miss my confidence in her
I miss her watchful eye on the future, unwilling to wait for 10x more

Blatant, pompous, physician's assistant, may Karma come knock at
your door

Vast

Overwhelmed by the tedium of doctor's offices
Hours wasted
Wait to be seen for answers
Shaded, smoke-filled with uncertainty
Leads to more appointments
More tests
Inconclusive vast answerless mess

Numbers

I felt my body bent
The burden of healthy heavy
Obnoxious in the intrusion
That comes so often
This winter so hard
To even admit relates the depth
Cruel fever and chills
No warmth
Sleep upon restless sleep
No blood pressure
Doctor upon doctor
So neatly arranged in February
Strung out 6 weeks, 3 months, 4 months, 4 weeks
Endless dates, co-pays, waiting
Illness, chairs, rows, dim lights
Paper-covered furniture
It is a hurry and a wait
Needles, more needles
Soaks up the deep red, labeled marked tagged
Answers with positivity
Assertively missing
Definitions of inconclusive, real
Felt
With each email release
Information in grey
I am grey
A ghost of uncertainty
Numbers on the edge of normal
percentages, decimal points of numerals unexplained

Infinitives

Doctor appointment
To new doctor appointment
To tests
To results
To wait
To wait
(1x2)1
To new directions
Serious implications
To wait
To new doctor
To old doctor
To cancelations list waiting
To new medications success
To prior authorization
To no
Rejection
Start again
To wait

Obsessing

Pent up feelings of madness?
Taken out on doctor?
Or body's doctor?
Taken out on patient?
Second guess symptoms
Move through house
A shell, a silent walker, lost in self
Second-guess, think, scheme
Relive imperfection, strive for perfection
Hold on with clenched jaws and teeth
Hold on to the meat of it
A situation finished, rewinds, replays in mind
Till corruption takes hold and the mind runs in circles
Rumpled hair
Lost feathers
And a stomach gurgles and intestines spasm
Perfection, perfection a race to nowhere
A known race
Unwinnable
And unable to stop doing it's done
Too much time spent, rehashing
Too much today lost
Too much numbing occurs in reckless haste
Too much over and over
And angry when over is interrupted
By loving friends
Obsession = me = doctor appointments = anxiety
I crave perfect healthcare
Paranoid if not
At the very bottom of it all afraid I will be worse, I will be sicker,
    I will die
And there is the real truth
Death is a fearsome thing
Disease is evil
Brings it closer? Ups the odds?
Complicates life? Scares you silly?

Release

How do you separate who you are from a disease?
When you are monitored 24 seven?
When a rope is about your neck?
When electrodes speed through the air?
The very information that will help you?
It does not help the mental part
But maybe yes?
A safety net as long as I am hooked up, someone is watching
Someone will know if I misfire again
Someone will just know period
Versus: maybe this or that
Or not very sure
This might be the worst
Indecisive doctors
Indecisiveness in this very word
Suddenly set free after 30 days
Freedom
From beeps and minutes
Thump against your chest sensors
Dying batteries beep beep beep
You're too far
Set free to remind yourself
You just might be normal

Searching Still

I am sad
Overwhelmed, doctor appointments
With indefinite conclusions
Blood draws, multiple vials later
Adjustments to pain
Bones out, then in, then out again
Blood tests I do not want
Cause stress in their very essence
Calls to remind me of appointments
While I am at appointments
EKGs not registered so taken twice
Text messages to appointment
Switching cars, movement just to drive to appointments
It is too much
Everything correlates to weight loss?
Stressed and sad
A blue day
A yellow sun day
Hot humid 90 day
Search solutions jockey organize
Schedule children husband
Infection
Flipped upside down world
And I am swimming backward, blindfolded

Not Even Here

All down
Comes from sickness
That I have had
From appointments
Running the maze
Circles lost
Tired rage, no energy
No anything
Negative negligent
Not even here
That could be the worst

Frail

Bitter frail
Body care
Over again and repeat
Appointments, schedules, tests
Needles times three
Bruised skin, results
Pain
In mind, in body, in soul
My soul hurts
Sore from it all, head wracking inexplicable
Adrenal glands, new lands
Prescription times
Trust in doctor, medicines, tests
Take the pills, hope for best
Unable to understand the significance of it all
Once
It was done
It was easily answered
Now
To remember the list? I cannot
It is long complicated
Layer stuck upon layer in crooked lines
I can't figure out
To describe this, which relates to that
And is connected through those
Does anyone really want to know? Not really
I barely know myself
It is bitter, it makes me frail
My mind cannot comprehend

New Diagnosis

And the grief begins anew
New diagnosis
And to what is the significance?
I do not know
Knowledge surpasses me, tumbles over me
Drowns me
A prefix of letters
A failed test
To now, a second opinion
Blood-work again
Again
Wait
Fast
Again
Arm is sore deep muscle sore
Spirit is manic, hysterical, sarcastic, manic
Partial diagnosis
Partially working
My mind goes knocking on another door
Reprieve
Conclusion
Look outward, miles away hilltops
Expressionless, lost
Frozen eyed distance
Time stills, unmoving am I

Electronic Research

A circle of impractical webbing
Drives knowledge away and toward
Confuses, illuminates
Craves more, more what?
Cure? Information? Reasons?
Answer correct and accurate?
Desperation drives crazy
Frustrations form the ring
The mind whirls about
Faster faster still
Until collapse takes over
And knowledge weeps down the side
Spills wide and is lost

Processing

It's a journey through doctor appointments and tests and tests
That lead to more
Afraid of new doctors afraid to look further
Because further is always found
And that leads to more
Needles in arm
In arm again
Bruised
Tired colorless
Wore out pair of work jeans
Faded light shine through reaching nowhere
The cloth is so thin
Does it filter the light and protect?
Or are the rays burning through its fragmented film?
I am the constant this body
This one miraculous body
Me cheeks flush
Think disease
Flush again
Fatigue nap learning curve sharp and changing
As to what can be done, accomplished
The body hides her curve protecting it, leaving the mind to wonder
Irritations springs at any disturbance
Not of her choosing
Away the look told
The control a farce, the way unknown
Tripping on the change of summer
Following rules of medication
Scared by the quantity
Wonder at the validity
Angry at the new diagnosis
Label of sorts
The shock suppressed by doctors so many
So many more
In the telling a piece lifts
Flakes off
Shrug off

Shake the excess
Downy fluff to breeze
Release me

Away She Runs Inside

Business, constant movement, practice
Brain spinning, words forgotten, misplaced, mis-said
Wrong word here and there
Correct, corrected, irritation
Remember, medicine, no clenching, eat right
Drink water, medicine, rest enough, eat well
Movement, medicine, bed sleep/no sleep
Who is to say?
Puzzled, scattered, mind inside
Eyes open, unseeing, unaware
Blink
Present in an instant
Where does she go?
Away she runs inside
Away she falls to fly
Lost in her thoughts of self
Lost to herself
Lost in her diseased host body, transparent
Whirl away
Frayed
Spring breeze blowing

Comply

Be an advocate
Don't be
Gain medical knowledge
Close your eyes and trust
Trust in things foreign
Unspeakable syllables a language unknown
Trust in education and strength of others
Comply with handfuls of medication
Doctoring unimaginable situations
Illiterate in the art form of the pills
Relinquish the responsibility
Closed
No more
End

The Pills I Swallow

I am the pills I swallow
Blue and red
And white
See through no color
Lemon yellow
White
A cocktail
Rich in helping?
A cocktail
On the run
Moving onward
Out
The pills I swallow, am I

Treatment

Monitor, treat
Treat to maintain
To manage
Ugly sweet cure
Where are you?
Unattainable imagination
So high, out of reach
Hands search out fingers flayed
Grasp anything
Nothing there, air
I do not look too far ahead
Too many medicines
Too many visits, lists, appointments
Filled
Full
Opinions, thoughts, guess
Subplots of intellect
Over educated
Forgot
Caught painted red
2 inch roller stripe
Ear to ear
Prickled headed unannounced flush

Check

New medications to take before bed
Stomach x2
Yeast x1
Eyes x1
Allergy x1
Just want to sleep
Feet stiff sore
Yet onward march out
Glass water more
Check, check
Medications started and selected
Yes, I medicated myself today
Check, check and check

Cautiously Optimistic

Pulsing headache
Runaway confusion
Emotions change by second by hour by day
Change one medication for another
Amusement ride of feelings
Physical psychological
Change
4 days till the headache is attributed to change
2 weeks psychological mudslide
Energy at 3 weeks doing moving going
Or is it sunlight, green grass and birds?
'Cautiously optimistic' a slogan
Political banner in nightmare of health
A new organ system under fire
A complex one, an engine sensitive to touch and timing
Stumble fall slow day
Slow because done so much?
Slow because new medicine doesn't work?
And blood-work normal
Bottom normal, absolute bottom normal
After having been on for 7 days
Everyone missed, with hindsight 20/20
Does everyone talk? Share? Communicate?
Joints inflamed once more
Move with care, walk with stiffness
Slow unbending bodily burden movement
Eyes swollen leak, weep upon waking
So much change so little information
10x4x10x1 daily
Blue, pink, white, tan, white
Coral oblong, half-moon circle
I observe, evolve
Comply

Cannot

I cannot begin to express how exhausted I have become
Dealing with this myriad of health unpleasantries
Medications keep reproducing
My palmed hands keep excepting
The bill grows and grows
I have no cash to pay
The sun does not shine
The moon is clouded past
The sky cries
The dried-up ducts of mine cannot

Conflict

The drum beat of medicine
Marching through the heart
Taking medicine for medicine for disease
Treat side effects for side effects from medicines
Where does it end?
People quit taking their medicine, I see why
It's exhausting set of hoops to climb over, under and around
It seems endless, thankless
And the side effects, treat this! Cure this! Cause this!
Sometimes I want others to literally be me for a week
And then see how they feel
If they feel too much
Or it they whine about little things
Or if they have any sympathy/empathy left at all?
It sucks away my feelings leaving residual rust covered anger, rage
Bitterness me
I don't want this
I'm tired
Fatigue the enemy
Paper thin skin
Sun burns daily
Hurt by words
Hurt
Hurting still

Distress

Panic

Don't let them see
The panic that is me
Oh yes there it is
SEE!
No smile, nod, hide
Easier? To pretend? There is no end to this chorus
Circling, tripping
Spinning down
Notice me- ME, forget me
Sick/healthy
Tired/full energy
Sad/Oh so happy!
Exhausting exchange of back and forth
Read me, past the facade
Look deeply and see
Save me from myself
Give me rules and structure
That I don't want
Love me regardless
Keep me close to heart
Imagine the great complexity of me
Creative, writing me acknowledge
Successful, smart me
If I am open
It hurts judgment of less intelligence
Less energy
Less strength
LESS PAIN, rejection
To admit to forget, to hurt, to tire, to fatigue, to body changing
Gaining weight, losing strength
Craving toxicity in comfort foods
Admitting too less is so painful
I hold my breath and will it away
Caught tight, caught needle of closed eye
Defeat
Chin up create parallel reality of
Fine

Energetic super productive opposites
To allude the hurt

A Disillusional Song

I have a Swiss cheese brain
Thoughts and words slide through and about
In illusive spirals I know nothing about
I laugh at its amusement
An almost uncontained crazy laugh
Where leaves become jumping frogs in roads
On a rainy Autumn night
I begin a thought with exclamation!
To be side tracked by a song
To be saying what was it?
But now the thought is gone
Slid away in Swiss cheese land
Mushy soft and dull rank with odor
I close a door on my fingers
Now one is black and red rimmed
At the nail bed end
I burn my arm on the fireplace
Blisters, burning pain
Ice it through, bedtime
My arm is on fire, injury, insult, hurt
I do not sleep
I toss and turn
I am awake
I get up at 5:45, because
My thoughts are as tangled as the bedding
Woven between my legs
I am antsy, walking, driven
Flopping back in bed, up again
I make breakfast
And sandwiches for lunches
I am myself, I am not myself
I am a stranger caught in a mind, that is caught in itself
Thinking and not, dazed, yawning lack of sleep
Staring into space
Floating in a kitchen, sitting on a stool
Holding a warm cup of coffee trying to ground myself
What is this place of half thought?

That leads to bruises and scrapes?
That chases sleep away?
That broods a thought, uncaught?
A tangible body, an intangible mind
Drifting, yet caught like fog in a valley
Grocery shopping with a list
Thank heavens for the list
And if it's not on the list, it never was
Home to laundry and groceries sorted away
A few lines of a book
Lunch
And writing
To try and capture this murky land of a sharp mind gone dull
With holes
A sharp mind, sharp enough to notice the holes and scared, sightless
What does this mean?
Where does this road lead?
What am I capable of?
I do not trust myself
Does my family trust me?
Is my husband having more? More to do? To plan? To check off and list?
Is that the role of a caretaker?
Am I in need of a caretaker?
Yet I am the caretaker?
So I set to sea, in this hazy mind
Lack of sleep, medicated mind
Trying to hold tight to here and now
Yet the sea is strong with currents, opaque
That cloud the judgements, time and space
I feel half a person
Or half the person I was
Yet more of a person as a banging stomach attest to
Hypersensitive to change
In the midst of nothing but change
Hypersensitive to words
Words I cannot catch and use myself
Able to read
Fatigued
Scattered jumpy thoughts that make others seasick
In the very abruptness of their wake

I want to scream
I want to cry

I want to wake up and say goodbye
To have this be over
Finished and gone
To be me, healthy cured
A disillusional song

I was a teacher...

The smell of dust in lockers
Fresh waxed floors and silent shoes
Deep breath years of movement
Bulletin boards and ghosts of students past
She smiles as her keys jingle on her new ID and lanyard
No lights to save energy, cooler than the crushing heat outside
She breaths in and slowly out
She is floating happiness itself
A new job, full time, a classroom all her own
The water fountain rattles on, 1960's tiled walls
Old school, full of paper, chalk dust time
She glides down the hallway in well loved sneakers
Carrying a box of new belongings to her room number 102
She reflects just before the metal fire proof doors painted an angry
    daffodil gold
'I am home'
I am where I truly belong
I have never been so present so here so content
Everything smells delicious
Opportunities like gold foil stars
Her room, her desk windows open no screens
Fresh new teaching supplies
the smell of new plastic folders and books
Make her drunk on the rolling of R
Wonderful old fashioned black boards, perfect for student
    conjugation
The alphabet and this years theme- cell phones, flip flops, traveling
    to the sea
Foil palm trees, a paper one too. Maps and tagged countries, que
    habla Español
She carries a smile everywhere, hardly conscious that she does
It is a part of her being, let loose among school doors
The excitement of new thoughts, ideas, and facts to explore
Taught multiple times yet always a new view to see
Through the magical fresh eyes of her students

This is almost too painful to write

It makes me mourn
For I was a teacher
And it's funny when you remember back
You only remember good and surely there was bad?
But when you mourn you only see the perfect was
Despite the is

Haunted Poise

The poise of a teacher
What is that anyway?
It haunts me still
Are you a teacher?
Awkward
Looking
What?
I was
I'm not
No
Confusion
Humor, laughter
A trace of sadness
Go back
To healthy, minus lupus
Working teacher
Gone, long gone
And ok
Whimsical snapshot backwards
Blink
Here, present, mom

Stranger

Who is that face?
Who is that girl?
A heart beat felt, stopped
Hold my breath, pause
Moon shape, round
Cheeks high and swollen
Eye narrow creases
She did not realize
I did not know
Till the frozen image smiled back at me
Is this what people see?
Voices, thoughts, shout back to me from past conversations
"You don't even look like you"
"You don't look like the person I married"
Pieces of me break away
I am this fat faced figure
I want to yell no! Not today!
Leave!
She is here to stay
Staring back at me from reflections
Do people know me?
Am I lost?
I see the face of sickness
I see the face of steroids
I didn't realize
I really didn't realize preoccupied with everything else
It hurt when I smiled back at me
With a strange new face
I didn't choose, I didn't see?

No

Crashed identity
No holding walls
No understanding of boundaries
Just no
Just lost
Darkness creeps in
Between breaths too quick to count
Between heartbeats skittering, stopping, spitting and anger hovers in
    warlike
Preparation
There is nowhere to run
Everywhere to fire
These thoughts unable to even grasp
These words skip as bad as heartbeats
-Stop-
Just no

Dripping with Fear

Write it out
Hash it out to purge
The dark matter of soul
The worry, the angst
The unsettled nature of I
To remember what has been able
Has been done
Not everything checks off a list at end of day
Some carry over and over perhaps to begin again
The dealing goes mad
And wavers at the steep pile of the to do, to get done
Finish accomplish see successful help
Time, time running
Fast swiftly by and fear staring eyes wide open fright
Filled fast longing for the peace
The happy
Ending beginning again
Mind filled with dreams of vacations
Away
Visiting every image a dream dreamt raptly
Wishing
Wishing hard for different views with no phone calls
Insurance doctors
Results medications rejection
Changed schedules medications
Identifications
New ones made appointment leading to new appointments
Too scary diagnosis?
The future drips with fear as day closes and shadows take the world
    by storm
Light ends and so leaves the mind

I am Lost?

The smell of fear
My disease and me
It closes in and I fall
I get back up
I limp
I limp and quick catch myself, smile
Before fear stained eyes scream out, white flag surrender, failure,
    quit
Frozen unmoving eyes
Unwilling, unwanting to see, set limitations
But the body knows
And I slide deeper down
Running I fall down
Moving I fall down
Moving I drop the dish
Pasta, pasta everywhere, sliding
Yellow on rose cherry
I hit the curb times three
So consumed by the idea of disease
I am strangled, silenced
The words are silent in my mind
I am thinking nothing
I am seeing little
Curled up, feet and legs drawn up
Notebook held close to chest
Writing out invisible demons
Of mind bending realities
Of mine, of theirs
It has me and I am lost?
My pen runs dry
Empty gone
Fleeting

Spit

Write out the ugliness the sickness
Stealing the soul
Write it out, spit it out every way but straight
Anger
What is it
What definition attributed by you?
Mad at wrong?
Mad at bad turns?
Mad at situations unsavory nature?
Mad at diagnosis
Which is part of me, but not me
Describes me, but isn't me
The juxtaposition is alarmingly frustrating
Severely lacking in terminology
Barely flattering at its best
Fierce fists ready crossed chest
Teeth clench
Squinted eye, eyebrows lowered
To fight what?
Yourself?
Letters on a page?
Label for a health insurance plan?
You are plastic sticky labels strung together
Wrapping body in garlands of tape
Angry at it all
Angry at none
It can't be undone
A new doctor, a new appointment, a new test
A new diagnosis, a new fear
A new hatred of circumstance
That may or may not be you

Unhinged

Wanting to shout
To scream unhinged cry
To run
Laugh like a mad woman
Curse like a sailor
This health
Is hurting me
Fearful killing me
Limits used up
Cashed in
Time elapsed gone
Disappeared
Fractured mind
Missing thoughts, words, deeds
Time of rest
Needed
Present moment soon
Half curved moon high

Hijacked

Wrong
Wrong word, right thought
Wrong
Lost
Lost word to thought
Judgment, laughter, hurt
Betrayed
Betrayed by mind and family, by mouth and brain judgment twice,
    to self, to body
Anger, black as tar, thick as sludge
Behind an angelic forced smile
Hatred in agreement
Hatred in joined laughter
Sadness
Grief
Betrayal, corruption, loss

Anger

I am full of anger
Rip you apart anger
Twisting through your body
Tangling rational thought
Clenched teeth angry
An anger that goes nowhere
And escapes everywhere
Or perhaps in my perfect world
I assume it goes everywhere
Even as I replay conversations or create future ones or change past
    ones
Anger paints my eyes black
And leaves them swollen, puffy eyed angry girl
With nowhere to run
Unable to run, able to scream
But that could scare someone
That could scare herself
Headache erupting
Depression descending
Anger chewing it all up
Shreds her very soul

Almost

I drown in next appointments
Next doctors
Next tests
I reach for light
Darkness descends
My turmoil has no end
My pool is full of nothing
Empty the vessel that is I

It is time to refill
Pour myself full
Yet I am lost in the how
The when
The where
Empty has no energy to move
To think, to begin

Empty is difficult
Hardness of steel
Fired to hot
Shattering strength

I look around to find
What?
The energy, the gasoline of go
Normal cures, no more
Almost to screaming madness
Almost to apathy
Almost, so close
A million miles gone

I am refilling broken
I am tired of the same
I am a suspended nowhere
I know that I am
I know not
Nothing, anymore done

Second-Hand Keys

Writing for life
For second-hand keys
That open to nowhere, nothing elsewhere, would be
Low, deep slow notes sung by
Cold fingers and toes
You want people to step inside and be you—a moment or two—then
    they might get it
Get you
Or get up and leave
This is the grey space of shadows and breath
Pulling you downward, angry in flesh
Base lull anger
Exhaustion in a house not your own
That morphs to blackness around you
From known to unknown
And the dream haunts you still so you wake up
Oh please wake up, you are safe
You are home

Three Six Nine

She didn't realize
6 months later, she didn't get it
This new thing with such a long name
Is here to stay
It doesn't go away, no cure
It's cause a convoluted answer
Caught on your tongue
Twisting your brain till it hurts
Its acronym, is hip, stylish even
No one has heard
I did not realize
I thought it passing nuisance
Treatable, curable, medicine able thing
But I am wrong
I listen to the doctor
Again take notes
Again
Loose words
Again
Leave
Again
The next day
It occurs to me
Research
And I do
I see the twisting answers
As confusing as my mind
Treatable, not
Diagnosis, not
So many unknowns
Not multiplied by nine
Another label for me
Another medicine to take every three
Anger anxiety
Anxious, nervous, dark
Inexplicable
Unknowing myself

Runaway thoughts
Caught by winter
Snowdrop promise

Thin

Thin as a whisper
Are the layers of me
Sleep elusive dream of heather
Mind a rave of notions
Thrown about
Haphazard
I am trying
To verbalize without the notion of romanticize
What is this epic
That is me?
It is not curable
It is subject in the fragment of thoughts
Of others
A guessing game of seconds
I wish not to play

Nostalgia

She doesn't remember herself anymore
She can't see past the new
She doesn't remember who she was before she was sick it has been
    so long
She has forgotten
Life without fatigue
Life short of breath
Running for joy
Running at all
She has forgotten her face free of rash
Apple round steroid face, swollen red eyes
Gone thick full crazy curly hair
Thin small shapely knees and ankles
Now swollen pouches fluid-filled and slowing
Down her knees and ankles
Erupting from nowhere, from everywhere
Heart flips flops, hiccups
And she is sad
Doctors more doctors
Medicines so many shapes and sizes
A mosaic of art
A toxic caustic art
That gives her back what movement she has
Four times a day by a handful at once
And then the fog settles in
Her words lost
She, herself lost
And she has forgotten who she was
Before
Before all of this
And all she sees is now
And it frightens her

Falling Sideways

Angry up and down thoughts
Tired
Working against me
Keeping me inside
Inside as the cold grips outside
Hurting face and hands
Aching joints hand, hip ankle wrist
Pain stabs quick and flees
Or stays 10 beats of heart
To fly away to other places
Knuckles shoulder
The body falls sideways
To rest
The eyes close
Left arm extended
Away to safety
10 minutes to an hour
Ear on bicep
Fingers curled
Legs bent
Sleep

Fractured

Words cutting jagged on a page
Fractured quality of rhythm
Mind in shards of health unrelenting
Care practices, hard-wire connections
Dangle twisted without
Transmitting information
Deemed essential
Frayed wires, crumble in duress
I, my friend, am a mess

Emergence

Geometrical Relief

When did the test get skeptical?
The decisions rendered, questioned?
There was a time when it was not so and things seemed smoother
Pleasant rolling along
Uncomplicated destinations
Shocking deep trust should be lost
Permanent? Semi? Transient?
Why?
A place safe to question?
A mind so wrought by disease it suffers misfires that shatter around
Breaking the glass edge, geometrical relief?

The coastal sound unchartered
The sand dunes moving
The gruff exterior of the storm yells and barks orders
Do you correct its course?
Is everyone afraid?
Has this storm warn away so much?
The beautiful edges of color
Leaving only brown?

What causes this doubt?
This disbelief?
The doubt comes from sickness
Where there once was none
It appeared forever
Changing the scenery
Without asking
Pulling the rug
Blindfolded
Unseeing sought
If cannot trust this body
Whom to trust?
In behaving so badly
There is no trust to self
So how do- to others?
As the next is coming

Robbing
Stealing
Slapping the face
Hostile taking, always taking
You will give no more
Not without fight, not without withdrawal
Arms crossed, saving core
Isolating core
Safe and aching turn in
Darkness gaze corrupted
No simple trust in store
For self, for others
For beaches strewn with debris

A gamble not wanting to have played
The lose so deep it weeps the soul of she
How to undo?
How to change?
How to trust again?
Nothing is as it seems
Second guess it all?
Or jump right in feet first
Hold your breath eyes wide open see the ball blink
Live the fall
Live the trust
Will it
Drive it
Be it
Hold fast today
In storm tomorrow
Hold fast fingers entwined interlaced
Not to be undone

Management

Emotional pit
A mess
Paper wasp thin
Unable
Simply unable
Move forward with life's demands
Sees little
No sound
Murmurs, unclear images
Fear
Of side effects, death really
Life-saving; medicine
Or hastens anew, diseases
Cure- no cure
There is only management
Cold management
Deep sadness
Pain, soul-wrenching pain

Conversations

What are you supposed to do?
Say hi I am sick?
Oh, I have this?
Do you care what others think?
Does it matter what they think?
The only person with the answer is me
And I don't know myself
Sometimes yes
Sometimes no
I crave the understanding, I hate the label
I want the acceptance
I don't want any questions
Don't tell me of your cures, miracle procedures, one day wonders
Don't tell me you have the same thing as me
YOU DON"T
You don't know, will never know
What is me and Lupus
Your memory is not mine
Your cold is not mine
Your knees are not mine
Your age is not the same as me and my Lupus
Your heart does not beat like mine
Your GI track is not mine
You do not take my medicines
You do not KNOW
And educating you is exhausting, beyond really
Beyond my physical realm of even wanting to
Are there classes to educate them on disease?
How to talk with someone?
How to relate?
How to just be?
To listen, share believe?
Impatience thrives inside me
At your ignorance
Perhaps nothing you ever say can be correct
Perhaps I don't want it
Perhaps my anger leaps out at an easy target

You
How does this end?
What is my choice?
I cannot say
I do not know

Unsolicited Advice

They do not realize they do it
Offer ideas of alternatives
When this fight is confusing obstacles
Of heavy iron hitting engines
Each its own distinct pat
Chewing on the whole
Compare me to Lymes Disease
And I am appalled
Do not compare me to anything
And they know another Lupus
And yet another and another
Does this comfort me to know there are others?
No. Not today I think
Does the burden lighten?
No. Not this moment, I believe
It is not helpful
To offer the flip side in the extreme
I might as well eat cloud dust
Drops of sunshine
And wind flowers
Side B plays backward
Hurts my ears, my mind, my well-being

Irksome

Irksome the corrections for the wrong words
Irksome the grasping for the right word
One name for another
A fictional movie plant, instead of a tropical tree
Two locations two separate states
The obvious, unobvious
The watching correcting, am I five?
Do I need a sign on my shirt
'It's the lupus'
'I am lupus fog"
'Yes I know - wrong word being said'
'No, I am not an idiot'
'Yes, I have chronic illness...'
'Lupus is stealing my brain'
'Corrections equal frustration'
'Do not attempt to pre-filter my words'
Post filter, change, correct
Do me the favor and ignore
Jumbled up riddles of words, scenarios
It is causing no death
And in this chaotic party condition
My mind beats bird wings in my head
Because the body is different
Sometimes unresponsive
Yet I am living, here, contributing
Take this new self
This medical pharmaceutical self
That keeps going
Believe in me
Keep the repugnant corrections to yourself
Embrace that I am here at all

Battle of You

Shock

You inherited a million war planes
They are bombing you

Down

You slide, in pain, hurting, broken
Body parts cascading down

Sinking

Into darkness, covers your eyes
You do not see, all is black of night

Fight

A frightening bouquet of colorful pills, swallow
Appointments consume, kill nucleus of you

Landmines

Explode with force unwanted, surprise
Tricky, tree stump, mud, rock-strewn, barren hike
Complications of you

Up

Rejoice, you are here, you have arrived floating up
Jelly legs weightless on exertion arrive on top
You have become, more

Embrace

Yourself, all of self, even the little warriors
Of immune fighting you
Civil war will reign, yet hold tight, arms incircle
The beautiful battle of you

Cherry Blossoms

I need a vacation
A nest in the woods, at the beach away, yes away
A secret hideout to curl up my knees hug myself and hide
Till I'm right again
Till I smile and laugh again
Till I breathe again
I need a vacation with pink cherry blossoms cool pools of water and
    color

Her Gift

A health prognosis
Driven by multiple diagnosis
Each a jagged fraction of me
Hold the person
Help the person
Wrap her in your arms and listen
Wait, patience
Saver her soul, her situation
Offer no judgment, just sincere affection
The reward is her certain gift
Her unique filled loving devotion
The sparkle that is hers alone
It is still there
Through the fog, inconsistencies
Misspelled, misfired directionless words
That trip on her tongue
Would you rather her silent staring?
Or shall she join this mixed up pitch?
Offer her bubble of curiosity?
Smile giggle of possibility?
Decide
Or rather she shall decide
And you are left
With your own accountability
Stand up, own yourself
Defend yourself
Be
Live
Choose

Opening

Wanting to reach out but this voice inside
Inside
Locks up tight withholding me from them
From me
Not wanting this, why have I created this?
Side effects of medication, body running haywire?
Choice? Physical? Mental? No choice?
What is it that locks me up? Lockjaw, arm, hand nothing speaks
Reaches out, grasps, it is frozen
Pulled tight protecting this body of being from perceived
Falling
Apart
Adrift
River of calamity
River of illness
Taking taking, erosion
Eating the edges, all of it
Stealing the pieces
Watching them drop away
The career
The life
The movement
The voice
The meaning of the person
The pain flood debris tangled in hair pulling
I do not want to still be locked in
The initial flood has cleaned
Now just occasional storms muddy the water
But they clear
So why am I still unreaching?
Holding words at bay
Arms at bay protecting fiercely, blindly
Robbing myself of pleasure? Habit?
In the realization comes the relief
The mental choice to action
The mental driving the physical to move just that one inch
To begin the outreach, to bring in the love

To feel the tenderness again, to smile
Curl up
Warm body to warm body and be

Alive

There is no positive hurrah
There is no race won
Walked, climbed, run
Although
There is a day lived
A smile given
A laugh shared
A roll of the eye
A silly goodbye
Chilly toes in blue bowed slippers
A teaspoon of Autumn honey, in a cup of coffee
Clean laundry, neatly folded
The smell of warm dinner
A table set in mixed matched placemats
Fiesta table, one in each color
Green plants, sunny room
A day given
Poinsettia blooms,
There is no hurrah
You are so happy in disease
You are never free
But you live on
Breath upon breath
Look about
Feel
See
Step
Here now
Alive

Popcorn Heart

Run away heart
Pitter patter fickle heart
Thump, skip, hop
Popcorn in the chest heart
Soldiers on
Dances on
Twirls in arcs of splendor

Remember the Important

What do I like?
Writing
Green plants
Water
Sea, pond, lake, stream
Movement, reflection of water
Reflected light, sparkles
The color purple
Blue, purple deep rumble indigo blue
Sunshine, sunset, sunrise
Sun on snow, sparkles
The quiet of Winter
The joy of Spring
The smell of Autumn
The sound of Summer nights
Floating in the sea on waves
Dreaming eyes closed outside on a righteous day
Silver blue pearls
Diamonds
Shards of light
Cherry pink wood
Books
Bookshelves full of books
Cats
Curled up with you chin on wrists sleeping
Flowers, all of them
Rounded petals waving intelligence, confidence
Knowing the answers why
Security, safety, love
Dark chocolate caramels
A brown leather belt
Cinderella movies
Comfortable undergarments
In bright shades of color
Alternative music that makes you feel
British humor
Romance

The movie *Hot Fuzz*
The book *Fault in our Stars*
Hawaii
Europe
Vacation
Toes skimming water on a dock
Cup and saucer coffee in hand on our deck at the cabin
Grey cat paw curled yawning
Sarcasm
True friendship
Smart husband
Good solid sons
Pelicans
History filled places
Old churches amazing stone architecture
Travel, the newness of it
Reading
The beauty of life
The pure
Physical nature about us, mother nature
In all her seasons
Zany printed shirts
Bright nail polish
Comfy jeans, girly dresses
Artful conversation
Floating contentment spaces
The journey of I

Shy Reaching

So foreign to herself
Closing doors she once held open
Why?
Is it a particular set of actions
She has become accustomed to?
To close off
Keep safe
The very little bit of self that had remained
Untouched
Uncorrupted by the disease
That has eaten her flesh
So many times
One becomes programmed to self-preservation
In harsh ways, incorrect ways
Until one knows better
Sees the bars
Not keeping others out
But herself in
Alone unmoving
Lonely
The thought turns to be
Open the door
Offer that shy smile again
Reach out
Look past
Remember love
Share yourself once more

Mostly

Mostly, my poems are happy
Mostly, I am happy
Or normal present in the swings of life
Good days, bad days
Lupus a series of health activities
Dealt with by day, by hour, by minute
It begs for attention, a deprived deranged puppy
And I am a cat person.

But mostly I am ok
The tar of toxicity, rarely grounds me long
I am moody at being stagnant
At being in this house
At being mired in sameness
I crave adventure and movement
New experience

But mostly I am happy
Or at the very least not as dark
Not drowning
Immobile, clawing inward
I am sitting on a porch in the shade of being
Out of doors being, seeing
Living freedom of summer giving
Not unhappy, not rejoicing

Being mostly happy
Still not consistent
Volatile moods
But mostly not so painted purple blue-black bruise
Rather a fair lavender grey

The Sun Comes Back

When a doctor appointment is slightly off
It reinforces that helpless
Oh my gosh feeling
That my disease is beating me, controlling me etc.
That I am in its throws and there is no escaping- unrealistic, of
    course
Yet in this twisted space it reaffirms this dark way

Breathe

Today the sun slowly peaks out, and blue sky emerges
As the rain grey front pushes East and away
The ground squishy wet tracks
Down comforter on the clothesline moving to the warming up day
And it is a new space
The disease is not that impossible darkness
It is just passing storms along the horizon
The sun does come back

You Will

I am not sure where the strength comes from
Many would categorize and file a name for it
I will not do that just yet
But deep within me holding fast is strength
Calling softly, you will manage the pain
You will manage the sickness
You will manage this disease
It travels up, in relation to any direction
Up to take that one more step
Up to smile amidst the uncertainty
Up through the chest around the heart and up
Is it nature-inspired?
Deep moist soil-driven?
Strength needs solid mass
Physical attributes
Something to hold on to during the cold gales of autoimmune disease
It is derived from a sisterhood of past powerful matriarchs
Motherless mothers to shelter?
It is female in nature as it relates to my very being
Courage high chin
Fire cat-eye determination
And I am grateful

The Simple Two

Ragged moods
Dash in and out
Through my tattered brain
Worn so thin form the basics of medical care
Run wild with disease
Awareness of the situation dawns slowly and illuminates
Erasing away unease
In the knowledge of
Faith returns
Hope peeks around the corner and decides to stay awhile
The body's shoulders drop
The jaw pauses
A smile for no reason
Brief but exists
To keep in this grain of irritation
And create that beautiful opaque sphere
So it doesn't hurt
Rub raw, bruise, the inner soft body
Perfect
The jewel strewn iridescent being of you
Transform slowly forward
Reach out
Pour over
Retain yourself
The bitter new
The precious old
The simple two

Edible Color

Each forward inclination is driven
By medically saturated intervention
And something else

Sweet southern wild flower breeze
Crickets singing praise to early August weather, returned again
Bright sunlight that crinkles the corners of eyes in delight
Soft hand to eyebrows, fingers cupped catching the warm yellow light

It is all rather cyclical
Flares of sunburst eruptions of disease
Milligrams of colors four times a day to appease
Humid smokey air
Green so many shades, avocado, fresh cabbage, deep sweet potato vine,
Edible string bean, carrot-topped feather joy

Birds everywhere intermingled with children's unhindered glee
Warm bare toes wiggle
Back rests gently wicker chair
Cool water ice cubes condensation slides
Head tilts back
Lazy eyes take all of this bounty in
Replenish the dry soul
Restore the wounded body
Healing in the green of summer

Bloom

Orange bloom in Pennsylvania
Out of setting, context
White petal fragrance
Enticing hummingbird love
Globes of orange simultaneous
Sweet scent points the nose to wind to direction driven
As out of moment as me
As out of place as I
Bearing fruit and the flower of possibility
Growing in shabby rock creek bottom soil
Transplanted to thriving loving opportunity
Proper soil, light, hydration
Nurture soul, body, imagination
Rise up tall
Face upward
Hear
Sit, crawl, rise again
And continue on hard work
Reconstruction starting at one
Girl unhinged, unbound, soaring jagged ruin fall rise
Reach out new
Hold tight bloom
Wind gust, take flight
Fingers of curls leading
Watching lemon cocktail purple flower
New growth driven in the thickness of summer

Lupus Fading

Lupus fading up
Blue turquoise opaque
White mist
Protruding from the center of me
Its weightless wonder
Propels the force of me out
Freeing
I am not lupus
It is part of me
It is with me
It is not the whole of what defines me.
Irritating catty little friend, yes
Consuming everything all, no
The lupus is fading up
Outward fleeing
Curling whisping about
Tickles teases my skin
Leaves me buoyant once again

She

She likes sparkly things she dreams big
She believes she can she always would

She chose her pen name
Even got the pen to do it with
She doesn't want to conform
To anything, no set rules
She wants to run with water
Rolling seeping conforming to
Nothing and everything
Letting gravity take her along
And dictate her path
The nature way
Her way
She is full of grey
Grey eyes with blue so
Maybe water and sky
Not deep water, clear
Shallow water
Rolling across a counter
As a glass tumbles over
And sky?
Not deep blue sky
Light aqua sky with feather clouds
She is movement
Never wanting to settle for too long
She is change, she is happy for change

Forward

English rose
Butter rum word
History deep
Feminine propriety softly
Smooth curve of hip
Off-shoulder
Elegant slide of hand, stretch
Rich feeling color
Taste of brownie smell
Intoxication bloom
Seasonless flower known
So many times new
Deep abyss, non-surface thoughts
Mirror present face
Pure soul light
Aquamarine color
Hands together
Up
Spread wide
Tree motion
Curve of air half circle
I live
I go beyond
I turn
Smile forward
Capture blue-back to grey, eye seen
Forward

About Atmosphere Press

Atmosphere Press is an independent, full-service publisher for excellent books in all genres and for all audiences. Learn more about what we do at atmospherepress.com.

We encourage you to check out some of Atmosphere's latest releases, which are available at Amazon.com and via order from your local bookstore:

A Synonym for Home, poetry by Kimberly Jarchow
The Cry of Being Born, poetry by Carol Mariano
Big Man Small Europe, poetry by Tristan Niskanen
In the Cloakroom of Proper Musings, a lyric narrative by Kristina Moriconi
Lucid_Malware.zip, poetry by Dylan Sonderman
The Unordering of Days, poetry by Jessica Palmer
It's Not About You, poetry by Daniel Casey
A Dream of Wide Water, poetry by Sharon Whitehill
Radical Dances of the Ferocious Kind, poetry by Tina Tru
The Woods Hold Us, poetry by Makani Speier-Brito
My Cemetery Friends: A Garden of Encounters at Mount Saint Mary in Queens, New York, nonfiction and poetry by Vincent J. Tomeo
Report from the Sea of Moisture, poetry by Stuart Jay Silverman
The Enemy of Everything, poetry by Michael Jones
The Stargazers, poetry by James McKee
The Pretend Life, poetry by Michelle Brooks
Minnesota and Other Poems, poetry by Daniel N. Nelson

About the Author

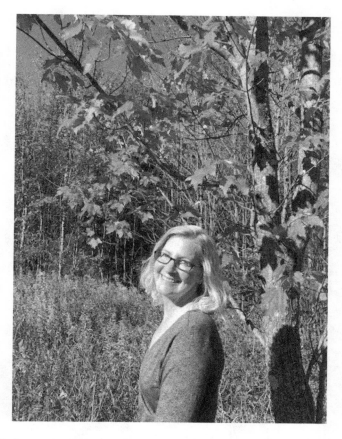

Tricia Johnson is a poet wishing to share her work with others, by using the written word to embrace one another's humanity. She is a retired teacher. She lives in the beautiful hills of Pennsylvania with her husband and two sons. Published work includes the poem "Living with Lupus" which appeared in *Still You Poems of Illness & Healing,* Wolf Ridge Press 2020.